IRIS MONTE

# The Fabulous After Fifty Handbook

*Empowering Lifestyle Strategies for Health, Vitality, and Radiance*

This book was professionally typeset on Reedsy.
Find out more at reedsy.com

# Contents

# Introduction

As you traverse the transformative journey of life beyond fifty, you may encounter a myriad of physical, emotional, and hormonal changes. These shifts, while daunting, are a natural part of aging. Nearly 75% of women experience significant health adjustments after this milestone age, highlighting the inevitability of these changes and underscoring the importance of understanding, accepting, and adapting to them.

Scientific exploration reveals the far-reaching impact of these changes on your energy levels, metabolism, and mood. Hormonal fluctuations can lead to decreased energy, altered metabolism, weight gain, body aches, and mood swings, affecting your daily life and overall well-being. However, with knowledge comes power. Understanding the science behind these transformations enables you to make informed choices to live a healthier, more fulfilling life.

Adopting targeted, sustainable lifestyle changes is crucial to navigating these challenges. Consider this: What if the next decade could be the best of your life? What shifts would you make today to secure your health and happiness tomorrow? This book invites you to reflect on your experiences and evaluate the steps necessary to embrace aging with grace and vitality.

Experts in women's health, such as Dr. Smith, a leading nutritionist, emphasized that "the choices women make in their fifties set the stage for the rest of their lives. It is never too late to embrace a healthier lifestyle." This guide's grounding in evidence-based research and professional insights ensures confidence in this advice.

Within these pages, five fundamental areas are the foundation for achieving long-term health and vitality. Each area, discussed in detail across five chapters, offers practical advice and actionable guidance to support you in navigating this new phase in life. This holistic approach addresses hormonal impacts on health, nutrition, physical activity, sleep, and stress management. Below is a brief overview of the primary topics for this book:

## 1 - Understanding Hormonal Health

- The role of key hormones in overall health
- Strategies for balancing hormones naturally
- Foods and supplements that support hormonal health
- Bonus Resource: Hormone-balancing foods chart

## 2 - Revitalize Your Diet

- The benefits of anti-inflammatory and nutrient-dense eating
- Optimizing macronutrient intake and hydration after 50
- Tips for stable energy and blood sugar levels
- Bonus Resource: A 7-day hormone-friendly meal plan

## 3 - Move Smarter, Not Harder

- The importance of movement for metabolism, bone density, and muscle mass
- Types of exercises to prioritize
- Tailoring intensity to your fitness level
- Bonus Resource: Weekly workout schedule with beginner to advanced options

## 4 - Master Rest and Recovery

- The science of sleep and its impact on hormonal health
- Strategies for better sleep during menopause
- The role of relaxation techniques in stress reduction and recovery
- Bonus Resource: Sleep tracker and bedtime hygiene checklist

## 5 - Build Resilience through Stress Management

- Chronic stress and its effects on health
- Simple stress management practices
- The importance of social connections and personal boundaries
- Bonus Resource: Stress management tools suggestions

As you embark on this journey, consider your current lifestyle and the potential for positive transformation. With each page, allow yourself to embrace the opportunities this pivotal chapter of your life presents. The goal is not merely to add years to your life but to infuse those years with energy, joy, and purpose.

Welcome to a world where aging is an opportunity for growth, self-discovery, and steps toward better health and vitality. Together, let us unlock the secrets to thriving in this dynamic stage of life.

# 1

# Understanding Hormonal Health

Hormones are mighty messengers that shape physical and emotional well-being. Understanding how hormonal shifts impact the body is essential for navigating menopause with ease.

This chapter will explore the role of crucial hormones like estrogen, progesterone, cortisol, and insulin in your overall health. You will learn how these hormones influence your metabolism, mood, energy, and more. We will also discuss strategies for naturally balancing your hormones through diet, physical activity, sleep, and stress reduction.

## The Role and Effects of Key Hormones

Hormonal health is a critical aspect of overall well-being, influencing both physical and emotional aspects of life. Understanding how essential hormones function and impact the body can provide valuable insights into maintaining balance and promoting health as we age.

## Estrogen and Progesterone

Estrogen and progesterone are two central hormones that play significant roles in female reproductive health. Produced primarily by the ovaries, these hormones work together to regulate the menstrual cycle, prepare the body for pregnancy, and support various functions essential for female reproductive development. Estrogen is crucial for developing sexual characteristics and maintaining bone health, while progesterone prepares the uterine lining for potential fertilization and supports early pregnancy stages (John Hopkins Medicine, 2019).

Beyond their reproductive roles, estrogen and progesterone also significantly influence emotional stability. Changes in these hormones' levels, such as those occurring during the menstrual cycle or menopause, can lead to mood swings and emotional fluctuations. Researchers have linked these variations to the neurotransmitter serotonin, known for regulating mood and emotion. When hormone levels are imbalanced, serotonin production may be affected, potentially leading to mood-related issues (Campbell & Jialal, 2022). So, no, you are not going crazy.

## Cortisol

Cortisol, often called the stress hormone, plays a pivotal role in managing our body's response to stressors. Produced by the adrenal glands, cortisol helps regulate metabolism and energy levels, ensuring adequate resources are available to meet demands during stressful situations. This hormone influences various bodily functions, including immune responses and inflammatory processes, highlighting its importance in maintaining homeostasis (John Hopkins Medicine, 2019).

However, long-term elevation of cortisol due to chronic stress can negatively affect health. It can contribute to issues like weight gain, sleep disturbances, and impaired cognitive function. Understanding how cortisol works allows individuals to explore strategies to manage stress effectively, thereby reducing negative impacts on health (Campbell & Jialal, 2022). Chronic stress is especially not a friend in our later years.

## Insulin and Thyroid

Insulin is another critical hormone produced by the pancreas that facilitates glucose uptake in cells, playing a vital role in metabolism and blood sugar regulation. Proper insulin function ensures that blood sugar levels remain stable, supplying the body with essential energy (John Hopkins Medicine, 2019). When insulin sensitivity is reduced, as seen in conditions like type 2 diabetes, it becomes challenging for the body to control blood sugar levels, leading to serious health complications. Maintaining healthy insulin function is thus crucial for metabolic health and overall well-being (Campbell & Jialal, 2022).

Hormonal fluctuations have far-reaching effects on basal metabolic rate, mood, and sleep patterns. The basal metabolic rate, which dictates how many calories the body needs at rest, can be affected by hormonal changes. For instance, thyroid hormones significantly impact metabolism; if they are out of balance, they can cause metabolic rates to increase or decrease, affecting weight management and energy levels (John Hopkins Medicine, 2019).

Furthermore, shifts in hormone levels can result in mood swings and emotional instability. These fluctuations can be particularly pronounced during life stages involving significant hormonal changes, such as puberty, pregnancy, or menopause. Recognizing these connections emphasizes the importance of monitoring and addressing hormonal imbalances to support mental health (Campbell & Jialal, 2022).

## Strategies and Support for Hormonal Balance

### *A Balanced Diet in Whole Foods*

A balanced diet rich in whole foods can play a significant role in supporting hormonal function. Incorporating a variety of fruits, vegetables, nuts, seeds, and lean proteins into daily meals ensures that the body receives the essential nutrients it needs. Whole foods are packed with vitamins, minerals, and antioxidants, which are vital for hormone production and regulation. For instance, leafy greens like spinach and kale provide magnesium, a mineral crucial for managing stress hormones and promoting relaxation. Additionally, consuming healthy fats from sources like avocados, olive oil, and nuts provides the body with omega-3s, supporting brain health and reducing inflammation. Studies show that diets low in refined sugars and carbohydrates help stabilize blood sugar levels, thus preventing insulin spikes and crashes——a key factor in hormonal imbalances (Franziska Spritzler, RD, CDE, 2017).

### *Regular Physical Activity*

Regular physical activity is another cornerstone in maintaining hormonal balance. Exercise helps regulate weight, which is critical for balancing hormones like estrogen and testosterone. Exercises such as walking, cycling, or yoga improve cardiovascular and muscle health and enhance mood by releasing endorphins - natural chemicals in the brain that boost happiness. Research indicates that exercise reduces cortisol, a hormone related to stress, thereby helping the body manage stress more effectively (Johnson, 2018).

## Stress Management

Effective stress management is fundamental to hormonal health, particularly in modulating cortisol production. Techniques like meditation, yoga, and deep-breathing exercises are effective ways to manage stress and reduce cortisol levels. Meditation promotes a state of relaxation by focusing the mind on breathing and clearing away distractions, leading to decreased anxiety and improved emotional stability. Yoga combines physical movement with deep breathing, enhancing flexibility and calming the nervous system simultaneously. Meanwhile, deep-breathing exercises enable practitioners to slow their heart rate and lower their blood pressure, creating a sense of calm and reducing stress-induced hormonal surges (Franziska Spritzler, RD, CDE, 2017).

## Superfoods and Supplements

Specific foods and supplements offer additional support in maintaining hormonal health by addressing nutritional deficiencies. Omega-3 fatty acids, found in fatty fish like salmon and mackerel, are known to support brain health and reduce symptoms of depression, a condition often linked to hormonal imbalances. Vitamin D, which can be synthesized through sun exposure or taken as a supplement, plays a crucial role in calcium absorption and bone health, and it has been associated with improved mood and immune function. Magnesium supplements may also help as they contribute to muscle relaxation and sleep quality, both important for hormone regulation. Adequate levels of these nutrients ensure that the body's endocrine system operates efficiently, promoting overall well-being (Johnson, 2018).

## Final Insights

By looking at essential hormones like estrogen, progesterone, cortisol, and insulin, we can understand how they influence different body functions. We also see how these hormones are involved in reproductive health, managing stress, controlling metabolism, and affecting mental health. We noted that changes in hormone levels can impact mood, sleep, and energy, so it is vital to recognize and manage these changes for overall well-being.

We looked at ways to keep hormones balanced through simple lifestyle choices. Eating a healthy diet, exercising regularly, and managing stress effectively can help support hormone function. We covered particular foods, exercises, and relaxation techniques that can aid in maintaining hormonal health, giving practical tips to improve well-being. By understanding how hormones affect their health, women can make better decisions about their lifestyle and promote a proactive approach to aging well. As a companion to this chapter, below is a food chart to assist in selecting hormone-balancing foods.

*Bonus Resource: Hormone-Balancing Foods Chart*

| Hormone & Focus | Beneficial Foods | Key Nutrients | Benefits |
| --- | --- | --- | --- |
| Estrogen Balance | Ground flaxseeds<br>Organic soy (tempeh, miso)<br>Pumpkin seeds<br>Cruciferous vegetables (broccoli, cauliflower) | Phytoestrogens, Lignans, Fiber | Reduces menopausal symptoms, supports bone health |
| Thyroid Support | Seaweed (kelp, nori)<br>Brazil nuts<br>Wild-caught fish<br>Eggs | Iodine, Selenium, Tyrosine | Maintaining a healthy metabolism supports energy levels |
| Cortisol (Stress) Management | Dark leafy greens<br>Avocados<br>Wild-caught salmon<br>Walnuts | Magnesium, Omega-3s, B vitamins | Reduces stress response, improves sleep quality |
| Insulin Balance | Cinnamon<br>Berries<br>Chia seeds<br>Lentils | Fiber, Antioxidants, Protein | Stabilizes blood sugar, supports weight management |
| Progesterone Support | Sweet potatoes<br>Chickpeas<br>Dark chocolate<br>Pumpkin | Zinc, Vitamin B6, Magnesium | Promotes sleep, reduces anxiety, supports mood |

## General Guidelines:

- Aim to include at least one food from each category daily
- Choose organic when possible to avoid hormone-disrupting pesticides
- Stay hydrated with filtered water
- Pair these foods with regular exercise and stress management

# 2

# Revitalize Your Diet

What you eat plays a central role in how you feel and age. Embracing an anti-inflammatory, nutrient-dense diet is vital to maintaining your health and vitality during menopause and beyond. In this chapter, we'll explore further the benefits of whole-food-based eating, how to optimize your nutrient intake after 50, and strategies for keeping your energy and blood sugar stable throughout the day.

## Understanding Anti-inflammatory and Nutrient-Dense Eating

As we age, our dietary needs change, and it becomes crucial to adopt eating habits that support overall health, particularly for those over 50. Anti-inflammatory and nutrient-dense eating emerged as powerful strategies in this regard. One key aspect of such a diet is focusing on foods rich in antioxidants, vitamins, and minerals, which can significantly reduce inflammation—a critical factor linked to various chronic diseases.

## Antioxidants

Antioxidants play a pivotal role in defending the body against oxidative stress and free radicals, which are unstable molecules that can cause cellular damage and inflammation. By incorporating antioxidant-rich foods like berries, cherries, and red grapes into the diet, individuals can help mitigate these harmful effects. These fruits are packed with antioxidants and provide essential vitamins and minerals that support optimal body function (The Basics of an Anti-Inflammatory Diet, 2024). Moreover, leafy green vegetables such as kale and spinach are excellent sources of vitamins A, C, and K, further enhancing their anti-inflammatory potential. Think of colorful vegetables when shopping for groceries.

Omega-3 fatty acids are another vital component of an anti-inflammatory diet. These healthy fats are known for their ability to reduce chronic inflammation, a common concern among those over 50. Omega-3s are predominantly found in fatty fish such as salmon, mackerel, and sardines; for those who prefer plant-based options, walnuts, flaxseeds, and chia seeds offer substantial amounts of these beneficial fats. The typical Western diet often contains an imbalance of omega-6 to omega-3 fatty acids, leaning heavily towards omega-6, which can promote inflammation. Thus, adjusting this balance by increasing omega-3 intake and reducing high omega-6 foods like certain vegetable oils can be advantageous (Zorn, 2023).

## Processed Foods

While bolstering the diet with anti-inflammatory foods is essential, reducing the consumption of processed foods is equally important. Processed foods often contain high levels of sugar, trans fats, and refined carbohydrates, all of which contribute to heightened inflammation levels. Cakes, cookies, chips, and fried foods are common culprits that should be limited. Instead, opting for whole foods, which are less likely to trigger inflammatory responses, can profoundly impact one's health (The Benefits of Eating an Anti-Inflammatory Diet, 2023).

## Phytonutrients

In addition to antioxidants and omega-3 fatty acids, phytonutrients deserve special mention. Phytonutrients are natural compounds also found in colorful fruits and vegetables. They are celebrated for their disease-preventive properties. Flavonoids and carotenoids have been shown to inhibit inflammatory processes and support immune function. Including a variety of colorful produce such as tomatoes, carrots, and blueberries in daily meals ensures a broad spectrum of these phytonutrients, each contributing uniquely to health.

The Mediterranean diet, a model of balanced nutrition that emphasizes omega-3 fatty acids, antioxidant-rich foods, and minimally processed foods, is a powerful tool in the fight against inflammation. By advocating for the consumption of olive oil, nuts, and lean proteins while discouraging the intake of red meat and processed foods, this dietary pattern has been linked to a myriad of health benefits. These include reduced risks of heart disease and improved longevity, making it a reliable and informed choice for those over 50 (The Basics of an Anti-Inflammatory Diet, 2024).

## Optimizing Macronutrient and Hydration Needs After 50

As individuals age, their nutritional needs evolve due to physiological changes and lifestyle adjustments. Understanding these altered requirements is crucial for maintaining overall health and vitality for adults over 50.

## Proteins

One of the significant changes involves macronutrient consumption, especially protein. Proteins play a vital role in sustaining muscle mass, which tends to decrease with age, leading to issues like reduced strength and mobility. Increased protein intake can support muscle maintenance and promote metabolic function. This is particularly important as older adults often face a decline in basal metabolic rate. Adequate protein can be incorporated into daily meals through various sources such as lean meat, poultry, fish, eggs, dairy products, legumes, and nuts (PMC8396619; National Institute on Aging, 2022).

## Healthy Fats

Alongside proteins, healthy fats are essential components of a revitalized diet. These nutrients aid in heart health and provide necessary energy reserves. Monounsaturated and polyunsaturated fats have been recognized for their benefits, including improving cardiovascular health and potentially reducing inflammation levels. Avocados, olive oil, nuts, and seeds are excellent sources of these healthy fats and should become staples in any diet designed for those over 50 (National Institute on Aging, 2022).

## Complex Carbohydrates

Dietary composition does not stop with proteins and fats. The inclusion of complex carbohydrates is another pivotal aspect. Unlike simple carbohydrates that may lead to quick spikes and crashes in blood sugar levels, complex carbohydrates provide slow-releasing energy, aiding in maintaining steady energy throughout the day. They are also beneficial for brain function, which can be particularly helpful in aging populations concerned with cognitive health. Whole grains, vegetables, and legumes are foods rich in complex carbohydrates that support long-lasting energy without the detrimental effects of simple sugars (PMC8396619).

## Fiber

Furthermore, fiber and hydration are two interlinked elements that must be considered when discussing diets for older adults. Fiber is crucial for maintaining digestive health, aiding in regular bowel movements, and preventing conditions like constipation, which can become more common with age. It can also help manage weight by promoting feelings of fullness, which is beneficial given the slower metabolism seen in older populations. Foods such as whole grains, fruits, vegetables, and legumes are fiber-rich and should be integral to daily eating habits (Li, 2016).

## Hydration

Hydration is a crucial aspect of health that often goes overlooked. As we age, our body's ability to conserve water and our sense of thirst diminish, making older adults particularly vulnerable to dehydration. This can lead to severe complications, including confusion, urinary tract infections, and kidney stones. Ensuring adequate fluid intake throughout the day is imperative. While individual hydration needs vary, a general guideline suggests aiming for about eight cups of fluid daily, accommodating variations based on activity level and climate. Remember, your health is our priority (National Institute on Aging, 2022).

## Final Thoughts

In this chapter, we have explored the essential components of a balanced diet that prioritizes health, particularly for individuals over 50. By incorporating antioxidant-rich foods like berries and leafy greens, we can reduce inflammation, which is linked to various chronic diseases. Additionally, omega-3 fatty acids found in fish and plant-based sources can further combat chronic inflammation common in older adults. We also highlighted the importance of balancing omega-6 and omega-3 intake, illustrating how dietary adjustments can promote overall well-being. By reducing processed foods in favor of whole, nutrient-dense options, we can significantly improve health outcomes, putting you in control of your health journey.

By gradually integrating these dietary practices, you can better navigate the challenges of aging with confidence and enhance your quality of life. As a companion to this chapter, below is a 7-day hormone-friendly meal plan to kickstart improving your diet.

### *Bonus Resource: A 7-Day Hormone-friendly Meal Plan*

| Day | Breakfast | Lunch | Dinner |
|---|---|---|---|
| 1 | Spinach and mushroom omelet with avocado slices | Grilled chicken salad with mixed greens, cherry tomatoes, cucumber, and olive oil dressing | Baked salmon with quinoa and steamed broccoli |
| 2 | Chia seed pudding with almond milk, berries, and chopped nuts | Lentil soup with a side salad and a small whole-grain roll | Stir-fried tofu with mixed vegetables and brown rice |
| 3 | Greek yogurt with low-sugar granola and sliced almonds | Turkey and avocado wrap with lettuce, tomato, and hummus spread | Slow-cooker chicken tikka masala with cauliflower rice |
| 4 | Scrambled eggs with smoked salmon, spinach, and whole-grain toast | Tuna salad with mixed greens, cherry tomatoes, and a light vinaigrette | Grilled shrimp skewers with roasted vegetables and quinoa |
| 5 | Overnight oats with almond milk, chia seeds, and mixed berries | Grilled veggie and hummus wrap with a side of carrot sticks | Baked cod with sweet potato wedges and steamed green beans |
| 6 | Smoothie bowl with spinach, banana, almond milk, and protein powder, topped with sliced almonds and chia seeds | Caprese salad with fresh mozzarella, tomatoes, basil, and balsamic glaze | Grilled tofu with stir-fried vegetables and cauliflower rice |
| 7 | Whole-grain toast with mashed avocado, sliced hardboiled egg, and everything bagel seasoning | Kale and quinoa salad with grilled chicken, cherry tomatoes, and a lemon-olive oil dressing | Baked tempeh with roasted Brussels sprouts and sweet potato |

**Note:** This meal plan focuses on whole, unprocessed foods, lean proteins, healthy fats, and fiber-rich options to support hormonal balance in women over 50. Remember to stay hydrated, limit caffeine and alcohol intake, and consult with a healthcare professional before making significant dietary changes.

# 3

# Move Smarter, Not Harder

Exercise is an essential component of healthy aging, supporting your physical and mental well-being in countless ways. However, the type and intensity of movement your body needs may change as you navigate menopause and beyond. This chapter explores how to optimize your fitness routine for lifelong health, focusing on low-impact exercises, functional strength, and activities you enjoy.

This chapter explores how informed movement choices improve health outcomes and longevity. Readers will delve into how different forms of exercise address specific health concerns such as bone density maintenance, muscle preservation, and cardiovascular support. This discussion includes evidence-based insights into the types of physical activities most beneficial for women over 50, highlighting ways to integrate these practices into everyday life effectively. Additionally, it explores the broader impacts of exercise on mental well-being and social engagement, emphasizing the holistic advantages of staying active. By focusing on personalized strategies that cater to diverse needs and preferences, this chapter provides practical guidance for adopting a balanced approach to movement, ultimately promoting a fulfilling and independent life as we age.

## The Comprehensive Benefits of Movement

Understanding how movement enhances overall health is crucial in today's fast-paced world, where maintaining a healthy lifestyle is more important than ever. One primary way movement benefits our health is by stimulating metabolism. Regular physical activity increases energy expenditure, which plays a vital role in burning calories and promoting fat oxidation. This metabolic boost helps in weight management, as it prevents the buildup of excess body fat, reducing the risk of obesity-related complications.

### *Bone Health*

Further, movement significantly supports bone health. Engaging in activities that require impact or significant load, such as light jogging, can enhance bone density and reduce the risk of osteoporosis, particularly in women over 50, who are more susceptible to this condition. Research suggests that running moderate distances, around 15–20 miles a week, is associated with maintaining or increasing bone mineral density (Warburton et al., 2006). This improvement in bone health is essential for preventing fractures and maintaining an active lifestyle as we age.

### *Muscle Health*

Regular exercise benefits bones and plays a crucial role in maintaining muscle mass. Maintaining muscle mass becomes increasingly essential as we age to prevent sarcopenia, a condition characterized by the loss of skeletal muscle mass and strength. Sarcopenia is commonly associated with aging and can significantly impact an individual's ability to perform daily activities. Engaging in consistent exercise routines that include resistance training can help preserve muscle mass and improve muscular strength, thereby maintaining functional independence into the later stages of life.

## Cardiovascular Health

Beyond muscles and bones, physical activity also contributes significantly to cardiovascular health. Exercise enhances blood circulation, ensuring that all parts of the body receive a steady supply of oxygen and nutrients. Improved circulation also means a reduced workload on the heart, which lowers the risk of cardiovascular diseases like hypertension, stroke, and heart attacks. Moreover, regular physical activity has been shown to reduce systemic inflammation, a key contributor to cardiovascular problems. The reduction in inflammation markers, such as C-reactive protein, directly correlates with decreased risks of chronic diseases (Warburton et al., 2006).

It's not just about keeping the heart pumping; exercise positively affects the vascular system, particularly the endothelium, the thin membrane lining the inside of the heart and blood vessels. Physical activity improves endothelial function, helping the arteries relax and allow increased blood flow while minimizing clot formation. This improvement can be seen even in people with pre-existing conditions, making exercise a powerful tool for managing cardiovascular health regardless of the starting point.

## Start Easy, Start Small

These physical benefits underscore why making movement a part of daily life is indispensable. Each type of movement, whether it's walking, dancing, or structured exercise like yoga or aerobic classes, contributes uniquely to overall health by targeting different systems within the body. For women over 50, incorporating varied forms of physical activity can be particularly beneficial, addressing age-related health challenges while promoting longevity and vitality.

While we delve into these specific areas, it's important to remember that any movement is better than none. Even small increments in daily physical activity can lead to significant health improvements. The concept of "move smarter" emphasizes quality and consistency over sheer intensity or volume. By tailoring activities to your physical abilities and preferences, you can create sustainable exercise habits that cater to your unique health needs.

Physical activity should not be viewed merely as an obligation but as a vital investment in one's future health. It should also be enjoyed. Integrating exercise into daily routines can transform perspectives; for instance, a morning walk can become a cherished time for reflection and connection with nature rather than a mere chore. You can also talk to a friend or family member while walking or even listen to a podcast or audiobook. If you are stuck at home, there are plenty of free online videos at your fingertips. Similarly, group fitness classes can offer social support and motivation, reinforcing positive behaviors and creating a community-oriented approach to health and wellness.

## Optimizing Exercise for Longevity

Embracing a well-rounded exercise routine is vital for extending lifespan and promoting overall health well into later years. At the core of an effective fitness regimen lies strength training, which plays a pivotal role in enhancing muscular strength and endurance. These benefits are essential for supporting daily activities and fostering long-term vitality. Maintaining muscle mass becomes increasingly vital as we age to counteract the natural decline that occurs over time. By incorporating regular strength exercises, individuals can improve their quality of life, reduce the risk of injury, and maintain independence.

## Strengthening

Incorporating low-impact strength exercises such as swimming and cycling can significantly enhance resilience while minimizing joint strain. These activities offer a gentle yet effective way to build stamina and endurance without putting excessive pressure on joints, making them ideal for older adults or anyone with joint concerns. Swimming, for example, provides buoyancy, reducing impact stress on the body while simultaneously offering a comprehensive workout that engages various muscle groups. Cycling, whether stationary or outdoor, encourages cardiovascular health alongside muscular development, supporting overall wellness.

Balance-focused activities like yoga and tai chi contribute immensely to improving coordination and stability. These practices emphasize controlled movements and mindfulness, which collectively help reduce the risk of falling, a significant concern as one ages. Yoga combines flexibility, strength, and balance, allowing participants to enhance their range of motion while calming the mind. Tai chi, with its gentle, flowing sequences, promotes stability and mental clarity. Both activities can be tailored to fit your abilities, ensuring accessibility across different fitness levels (Delfin & Delfin, 2024).

## Modify Your Activity

For exercise routines to be truly beneficial, adjusting intensity based on individual fitness levels and goals is critical. It's not just about what exercises you choose but how you execute them that determines their effectiveness. Tailoring intensity allows individuals to align workouts with personal capacities, ensuring exercises are challenging yet achievable. This approach prevents burnout, reduces injury risk, and supports sustainable progress over time. A good starting point might include moderate activities, gradually increasing intensity as strength and stamina build (National Institute on Aging, 2022). Remember not to compare yourself to others in group exercise classes. Everyone is at a different pace.

## Call To Action

Implementing a strategy that incorporates variation and adapts exercises as capabilities evolve is equally important. Flexibility in routines keeps the practice engaging and targets different muscle groups, thereby preventing plateaus. Tracking progress and celebrating milestones, no matter how small, reinforces commitment and motivation. Additionally, consulting healthcare professionals before embarking on new regimens ensures safety and appropriateness, particularly if physical limitations exist.

Engaging with community resources like gym group classes or community walking clubs can further enrich your exercise experience. Such settings foster social connections, provide accountability, and infuse a sense of camaraderie that also enhances motivation. Understanding that physical activity offers emotional benefits as well, many find participating in group settings elevates their mood.

## Summary and Reflections

The chapter has outlined numerous health benefits that intelligent movement can bring, emphasizing how these practices are particularly valuable for women over 50. From improving bone and muscle health to boosting cardiovascular function, regular physical activity is a key contributor to overall well-being. By engaging in tailored exercise routines, individuals can manage weight, maintain bone density, and sustain muscle mass—all critical factors in reducing the risk of age-related health issues. Furthermore, incorporating a variety of activities like yoga or tai chi ensures improvements in balance and coordination, adding layers of protection against potential injuries.

As a companion to this chapter, below are some suggestions for workout routines to jumpstart your activity routine.

## *Bonus Resource: Weekly Workout Schedule with Beginner to Advanced Options*

| Day | Focus | Beginner | Intermediate | Advanced |
|---|---|---|---|---|
| Monday | Total Body Strength | Chair-assisted squats (2x8-10)<br>Wall push-ups (2x8-10)<br>Seated band rows (2x10)<br>Standing calf raises with support (2x10)<br>Bird dogs (2x6 each side) | Regular bodyweight squats (3x12)<br>Incline push-ups (3x10)<br>Standing band rows (3x12)<br>Walking lunges (2x10 each leg)<br>Plank holds (3x20s) | Dumbbell squats (3x15)<br>Regular push-ups (3x12)<br>Dumbbell rows (3x15)<br>Weighted walking lunges (3x12 each)<br>Plank holds with leg lifts (3x30s) |
| Tuesday | Cardio & Balance | Walking 10-15 mins<br>Seated marching (2x30s)<br>Heel-to-toe walk (2x10 steps)<br>Supported single-leg stands (2x10s each) | Brisk walk/light jog 20-25 mins<br>Step-ups (3x12 each)<br>Tandem walking (3x15 steps)<br>Single-leg stands with arms (3x15s) | Interval walk/jog 30 mins<br>Weighted step-ups (3x15 each)<br>Agility ladder drills (3 sets)<br>Single-leg balance eyes closed (3x20s) |
| Wednesday | Flexibility & Recovery | Gentle yoga/stretching 15 mins<br>Hamstring stretches<br>Hip flexor stretches<br>Light walking 10 mins | Yoga/stretching 20 mins<br>All beginner stretches plus:<br>Shoulder mobility work<br>Walking 15 mins | Yoga/stretching 30 mins<br>All intermediate work plus:<br>Advanced balance poses<br>Walking 15-20 mins |
| Thursday | Functional Fitness | Sit-to-stand (2x8)<br>Counter push-ups (2x8)<br>Band pulls (2x10)<br>Step-touch (2x30s)<br>Bridges (2x10) | Squat to overhead reach (3x12)<br>Modified burpees (3x8)<br>Band pull-aparts (3x12)<br>Banded side steps (3x20)<br>Bird-dog planks (3x30s) | Kettlebell swings (3x15)<br>Full burpees (3x10)<br>TRX rows (3x15)<br>Lateral bounds (3x12 each)<br>Side planks with rotation (3x45s) |
| Friday | Cardio & Core | Seated punches (3x30s)<br>Seated knee lifts (2x30s)<br>Standing twists (2x20s)<br>Modified crunches (2x10)<br>Pelvic tilts (2x10) | Standing punches with weights (3x45s)<br>Step-outs (3x45s)<br>Standing wood chops (3x12 each)<br>Bicycle crunches (3x15)<br>Dead bugs (3x10 each) | Boxing combinations (3x60s)<br>Jump rope or alternative (3x60s)<br>Medicine ball rotations (3x15 each)<br>Plank to down dog (3x12)<br>Turkish get-ups (3x5 each) |
| Saturday | Active Recovery | Choose one:<br>Walking 20 mins<br>Light swimming<br>Gentle cycling<br>Light gardening | Choose one:<br>Walking 25 mins<br>Swimming<br>Cycling<br>Gardening | Choose one:<br>Walking 30 mins<br>Lap swimming<br>Moderate cycling<br>Active gardening |
| Sunday | Rest | Complete rest or light stretching | Complete rest or light stretching | Complete rest or light stretching |

## Track these metrics monthly:

1. 30-second chair stand count
2. 400m walking speed
3. Single-leg balance time
4. Modified push-up count

5. Sit-and-reach flexibility

**Safety Notes**

- Consult with your physician before starting a new exercise regimen or if you have physical or health limitations
- Stop if you experience pain
- Prioritize form over speed/weight
- Stay hydrated
- Wear appropriate footwear
- Exercise in a clear, well-lit space
- Keep emergency contacts handy

Progress to the next level when current exercises feel comfortable for 4-6 consecutive weeks.

# 4

# Master Rest and Recovery

Sleep and recovery are often overlooked in the pursuit of health, but they are essential components of your well-being. During menopause, hormonal shifts can disrupt your sleep patterns and energy levels. In this chapter, you will learn about the science of sleep, common sleep challenges during menopause, and strategies for optimizing your rest and recovery.

This chapter explores various aspects of restful sleep and recovery techniques that are particularly beneficial during menopause. It delves into the science behind sleep, emphasizing its role in hormone regulation and stress management. Additionally, the chapter examines common sleep disturbances faced during menopause and offers practical solutions, ranging from sleep hygiene tips to mindfulness practices. This chapter provides simple hacks for improving sleep quality. By adopting some of these strategies, individuals gain insights into fostering a healthier routine that supports their journey through menopause and beyond.

## The Science of Sleep and Addressing Disruptions

Sleep plays a pivotal role in regulating hormones, which is particularly significant during menopause—a time marked by hormonal fluctuations. During deep sleep stages, the body works to balance crucial hormones such as cortisol and growth hormone. Cortisol, known as the stress hormone, follows a diurnal rhythm that is typically low at night, allowing the body to rest and recover from daily stressors. Growth hormone, released during deep sleep, aids in cell repair and regeneration, essential processes for maintaining overall health and managing stress. By ensuring these hormones are balanced, quality sleep becomes a cornerstone of well-being during the transitional phase of menopause (Askinazi, 2023).

However, menopause often causes sleep disturbances, primarily due to hormonal changes. The decline in estrogen levels can lead to hot flashes and night sweats, both of which significantly disrupt sleep patterns. Many women report frequent awakenings throughout the night, leading to insomnia—a common menopausal complaint. These disruptions affect nighttime rest and can result in daytime fatigue, impacting mood and cognitive function (Nowakowski et al., 2013).

Addressing sleep issues during menopause requires a multifaceted approach. Implementing strategies like maintaining a consistent sleep schedule can help regulate the body's internal clock, making falling and staying asleep easier. Creating a relaxing bedtime routine also signals the brain that it is time to unwind, promoting a more restful sleep environment. Simple habits like dimming lights, engaging in calming activities, or taking a warm bath before bed can significantly reduce sleep disturbances.

## *Guideline: Creating a Sleep-Conducive Environment*

- Establish a regular sleep-wake cycle by going to bed and waking up at the same time every day.
- Create a calming pre-sleep routine involving relaxing activities such as a hot bath, candles, aromatherapy, reading, or listening to soothing music.
- Optimize your sleep environment by keeping the bedroom cool, dark, and quiet. If necessary, you can use earplugs or an eye mask.

Professional guidance might be necessary for those with severe sleep issues. Consulting with a healthcare provider can help identify specific factors contributing to insomnia and determine the best course of action. Strategies may include behavioral therapies, lifestyle modifications, or even exploring potential medical interventions. Seeking expert advice ensures that any treatment plan is personalized and considers all aspects of the individual's health and lifestyle.

## Enhancing Recovery Through Mindfulness and Sleep Hygiene

Mastering rest and recovery, particularly during menopause, entails understanding and adopting practices that cultivate restorative sleep and effective recovery. One foundational aspect is enhancing sleep hygiene, including creating an optimal sleep environment and reducing screen exposure before bedtime. This practice fosters better sleep quality and plays a crucial role in maintaining overall health and well-being.

Establishing a healthy routine can begin with evaluating one's sleep environment. A bedroom conducive to sleep should be cool, dark, and quiet, minimizing distractions and optimizing comfort. Investing in blackout curtains or white noise machines might create an ideal setting for slumber. Eliminating electronic devices, such as phones and televisions, at least an hour before bedtime can significantly improve sleep by reducing blue light exposure, which is known to disrupt circadian rhythms (Suni & Singh, 2023).

## Mindfulness Practices

Mindfulness emerges as a powerful tool for recovery, especially through regular meditation practices. For those navigating the challenges of menopause, stress reduction becomes critical for promoting relaxation and improving sleep patterns. Engaging in simple mindfulness techniques helps center the mind and alleviate anxiety. Whether through guided meditations, yoga, or tai chi, these practices encourage a calm mental state, facilitating smoother transitions into restful sleep (Comprehensive Guide to Sleep Hygiene, 2024).

Incorporating breathing exercises into daily routines serves as another complementary strategy. Activities such as deep breathing focus on intentional breath regulation, calming both the mind and body. Breathing exercises are particularly beneficial at bedtime, assisting individuals in winding down after demanding days. These exercises promote relaxation by triggering the parasympathetic nervous system, effectively preparing the body for restorative sleep.

Aromatherapy offers an additional resource for enhancing relaxation and sleep quality. Utilizing essential oils like lavender can create a peaceful ambiance and trigger sensory mechanisms that promote sleep. Lavender, with its soothing properties, has been shown to reduce anxiety and improve sleep onset when used consistently. Diffusing essential oils in the bedroom before bedtime or adding a few drops to a warm bath can nurture a tranquil atmosphere conducive to rest.

## Final Thoughts

In this chapter, we explored how restful sleep and effective recovery techniques can significantly enhance your well-being during menopause. We dug into the science behind how sleep regulates hormones like cortisol and growth hormone, which are crucial during this transitional phase.

Understanding the impact of hormonal changes on sleep disturbances, such as night sweats and hot flashes, highlights the importance of addressing these disruptions to improve overall health. Implementing a consistent sleep schedule, creating a calming bedtime routine, and optimizing your sleep environment are practical strategies you can use to combat insomnia and promote restorative rest. A bonus checklist is included below to help you get started.

*Bonus Resource: Sleep Tracker and Bedtime Hygiene Checklist*

| Task | Completed (Y/N) |
| --- | --- |
| Stick to a consistent sleep schedule | |
| Avoid caffeine, alcohol, and large meals close to bedtime | |
| Create a relaxing bedtime routine (e.g., reading, meditation, warm bath) | |
| Ensure the bedroom is quiet, dark, and at a comfortable temperature | |
| Use the bed only for sleep and intimacy | |
| Avoid electronics (TV, phone, tablet) at least 30 minutes before bed | |
| Get regular exercise, but not too close to bedtime | |
| Manage stress through relaxation techniques (deep breathing, journaling) | |
| If unable to sleep after 20 minutes, get up and do a calming activity | |
| Expose yourself to natural light during the day to regulate sleep-wake cycle | |

**Remember**:

- Consistently tracking your sleep can help identify patterns and areas for improvement.
- Implementing good bedtime hygiene habits can promote better sleep quality and duration.
- If sleep problems persist, consult with a healthcare professional for further guidance.

# 5

# Build Resilience through Stress Management

Stress is a natural part of life, but chronic stress can damage physical and emotional health. Hormonal changes during menopause can amplify the effects of stress, making it especially important to prioritize stress management. This chapter explores the impact of chronic stress, practical strategies for reducing stress, and the importance of building resilience.

This chapter explores the relationship between chronic stress and its detrimental effects on physical and mental wellness. It discusses the role of cortisol, a primary stress hormone, and how its excessive presence due to chronic stress can lead to suppressed immune function and increased susceptibility to illnesses. The connection between high cortisol levels and heightened risks of cardiovascular diseases is also discussed, highlighting the importance of mitigating stress to prevent heart-related complications.

In addition to physical health, the chapter addresses the impact of chronic stress on mental health disorders. It sheds light on how stress hormones influence neurotransmitter balance, potentially leading to conditions such as anxiety and depression. Furthermore, we discuss how stress exacerbates existing chronic conditions by intensifying

the body's natural resilience diminishes with age. Recognizing stressors and their impact can help individuals take deliberate steps to manage them effectively. By understanding how chronic stress influences the body's intricate systems, individuals can better appreciate the necessity of integrating stress reduction techniques into daily life. This is crucial for improving immediate well-being and enhancing the quality and length of life as we age.

## Strategies for Managing Stress and Cultivating Support

Navigating the challenges of stress is crucial for enhancing resilience and ensuring we can adapt effectively to life's ups and downs. One potent strategy involves mindfulness practices. Mindfulness promotes awareness and acceptance of the present moment, which directly contributes to reducing stress. This reduction occurs as mindfulness lowers cortisol levels, a hormone often linked to stress, thus improving emotional regulation. By focusing on the here and now, individuals cultivate an inner calmness that helps them manage stress more effectively.

### *Breathing Exercises & Gratitude*

As mentioned in the chapter on sleep, deep breathing exercises are another effective method of combating stress. These techniques activate the parasympathetic nervous system, counteracting the body's stress responses. Deep breathing exercises can reduce blood pressure and heart rate when practiced regularly. By focusing on slow, deliberate breaths, the body receives a signal to relax, moving away from the fight-or-flight response typically associated with stressful situations.

Gratitude practice is also invaluable in managing stress. Regularly acknowledging things you are grateful for fosters a positive mindset. This shift in focus not only improves mood but also strengthens interpersonal relationships. When people recognize and express gratitude, they tend to see improvements in their interactions with others, creating a supportive environment that can buffer against stress.

## Fostering Personal Boundaries

Establishing clear boundaries is vital in stress management. In to-day's fast-paced world, understanding where to draw the line between personal time and obligations can prevent overwhelm. By setting boundaries, individuals protect their mental health, ensuring there is adequate time for self-care, reflection, and relaxation. Alongside this, nurturing a reliable support system provides both emotional security and practical assistance. Having a group of trusted individuals to lean on can ease the burdens of stress, making challenges feel more manageable.

The importance of setting boundaries and cultivating a support system cannot be overstated. Boundaries act as a protective measure, preventing burnout and preserving well-being. Meanwhile, a strong support network offers a safety net, allowing individuals to share concerns and receive encouragement. Friends and family offer perspectives that can help reframe stressful situations, transforming them into opportunities for growth and learning.

A practical guideline for setting boundaries includes assessing one's limits and communicating them clearly to others. It is critical to identify what is non-negotiable in terms of personal time and commitments. Once boundaries are established, it becomes easier to say no to demands that encroach upon this protected space. Consistent reinforcement of these boundaries ensures they are respected over time.

## *Mindfulness Practices*

Just as was presented for improving sleep, integrating mindfulness, deep breathing, gratitude practice, boundary setting, and support systems can help individuals effectively manage stress and bolster resilience. Each method contributes uniquely to stress reduction and resilience building, collectively offering a comprehensive approach to sustaining well-being.

Incorporating mindfulness into daily routines can be as simple as short meditation sessions, focusing on breath, or mindful walking. The essence is to be present, allowing thoughts to flow without judgment. Deep breathing can complement mindfulness, serving as a tool to anchor oneself during moments of anxiety or tension.

Maintaining a gratitude journal is also beneficial. It allows you to jot down daily reflections on what you appreciate. Over time, this shifts attention from stressors to sources of joy and contentment, fostering a more optimistic outlook.

## Bringing It All Together

Understanding the impact of chronic stress is essential for building resilience. Just like sleep, we explored how stress affects both physical and mental health, highlighting its role in weakening our immune system and increasing risks for cardiovascular diseases and mental health disorders. By examining these effects, we recognize the importance of addressing stress to prevent further health complications. Strategies like mindfulness, deep breathing exercises, gratitude practices, and setting boundaries were discussed as effective methods for managing stress. These approaches are beneficial for immediate stress relief and crucial for long-term health and overall well-being. Below is a summarized list of stress management tools for easy reference.

# *Bonus Resource: Stress Management Tools Suggestions*

| Tool | Description | Benefits |
| --- | --- | --- |
| Mindfulness Meditation | Practice focusing on the present moment, observing thoughts and feelings without judgment | Reduces stress, anxiety, and depression; improves emotional regulation and self-awareness |
| Deep Breathing Exercises | Take slow, deep breaths from the diaphragm to promote relaxation | Lowers heart rate and blood pressure, reduces muscle tension, and promotes a sense of calm |
| Progressive Muscle Relaxation | Systematically tense and relax muscle groups to release physical tension | Reduces muscle tension, improves sleep quality, and promotes overall relaxation |
| Yoga | Combine physical postures, breathing techniques, and meditation for a holistic mind-body practice | Improves flexibility, strength, balance, and reduces stress and anxiety |
| Journaling | Write down thoughts, feelings, and experiences to process emotions and gain self-insight | Provides emotional outlet, helps identify stressors and patterns, and promotes problem-solving |
| Social Support | Connect with friends, family, or support groups for emotional support and companionship | Reduces feelings of isolation, provides a sense of belonging, and offers different perspectives |
| Time Management | Prioritize tasks, set realistic goals, and create a balanced schedule to manage responsibilities | Reduces feelings of overwhelm, increases productivity, and allows for self-care and leisure time |
| Hobbies and Leisure Activities | Engage in enjoyable activities like reading, gardening, or crafting to unwind and recharge | Provides a mental break from stressors, promotes creativity and self-expression, and boosts mood |
| Physical Exercise | Engage in regular physical activity like walking, swimming, or dancing for stress relief and overall health | Releases endorphins, improves sleep quality, boosts energy levels, and enhances mental well-being |
| Professional Support | Seek guidance from a therapist or counselor to develop coping strategies and address underlying issues | Provides personalized support, offers new perspectives and skills, and promotes emotional healing |

## **Remember**:

- Different tools may work better for other individuals and situations.
- Consistency and regular practice are key for maximum stress relief benefits.

- Feel free to seek professional help if stress feels unmanageable or overwhelming.

# 6

# Conclusion

## A Fabulous Path to Better Health

Starting a journey towards better health means making thoughtful changes that last. Quick fixes and extreme diets usually only work in the short term. Instead, small, evidence-based changes to daily habits can significantly improve overall health. This approach focuses on immediate benefits while building healthy habits for life. By concentrating on sustainability, people can easily fit healthier routines into their everyday lives, creating a balanced lifestyle.

In the previous chapters, we examined five important areas supported by research, each helping to improve health. We discussed the importance of understanding hormones and improving diets. We also talked about staying active, getting good sleep, and managing stress. By examining how these changes work together, we found they support overall health, especially for women over 50. Making these changes can lead to significant health improvements, helping women feel energetic and strong in their later years.

## Consistency and the Long-Term Roadmap

Adopting a sustainable health approach requires intentional, incremental actions supported by a commitment to enduring change. It is crucial to understand the importance of starting small and slow. By setting realistic goals, you can remain consistent without feeling overwhelmed. This gradual strategy is rooted in behavior change theories, such as the Fogg Behavior Model, which emphasizes that simplicity is essential for developing habits. Pursuing overly ambitious changes can lead to exhaustion and disillusion. Concentrating on one attainable goal at a time builds confidence and sets the stage for additional improvements.

Psychological factors play a vital role in sustaining lifestyle changes. Developing positive habits and fostering internal motivation are essential for lasting transformation. New behaviors become ingrained when they become routine, thereby reducing the mental effort required. Intrinsic motivation—driven by personal fulfillment—promotes more extraordinary dedication than external pressures, such as societal expectations. Understanding these psychological dynamics is key to developing healthy habits and strengthening the resolve to maintain them.

## *Challenges and Setbacks – Assess, Modify, and Continue Forward*

Encountering challenges and setbacks is a natural part of the process. You may frequently face hurdles that threaten your progress, whether due to time limitations, lack of resources, social pressure, etc. Insights from behavioral health research provide practical solutions. For instance, breaking down larger tasks into smaller, manageable steps can make daunting objectives feel more achievable. Learning from the success stories of others who have overcome similar difficulties can reignite determination by giving you new ideas and motivation. Utilizing problem-solving techniques, such as identifying triggers and creating contingency plans, empowers you to address potential obstacles effectively.

## Strategy for the Future

Regular self-assessment celebrates accomplishments while identifying areas for development. Maintaining adaptable plans is particularly important as life circumstances evolve. Modifying exercise regimens and dietary habits to match age and physical capabilities helps prevent stagnation and sustains your motivation.

Establishing a flexible plan is crucial for long-term advancement. This includes setting realistic expectations, recognizing and celebrating milestones, and routinely reevaluating goals to ensure they align with personal aspirations. It is important to acknowledge that progress may vary; successes will accompany challenges. Remaining adaptable in the face of unexpected situations allows you to keep your focus on overarching health objectives.

## Final Thoughts

I hope this book has illuminated the profound impact that sustainable lifestyle changes can have on the health and well-being of women over 50. By understanding the power of these choices, you can approach the journey of integrating healthy habits into your daily life with renewed motivation and clarity.

The key to success lies in starting small and maintaining consistency over time. As you navigate this path:

- Embrace the power of self-awareness and adaptability

- Regularly assess your progress
- Celebrate your wins!
- Acknowledge your strengths and areas for growth
- Be willing to adjust your approach as your circumstances and needs evolve
- Always keep your well-being at the forefront

Throughout your journey, surround yourself with a supportive network, and do not hesitate to ask for help when needed. Building a strong foundation of social connections can be a powerful catalyst for positive change and a source of joy and resilience.

Please remember to consult with your doctor before making any significant lifestyle changes. This will ensure that your journey towards better health is safe, effective, and tailored to your circumstances.

As you embark on this transformative path, embrace the power of small, consistent changes and trust in your ability to thrive. May this book be a source of inspiration, guidance, and empowerment as you navigate the beautiful journey of life beyond your fabulous 50s. Cheers to a future filled with joy, resilience, and the radiant glow of a life well-lived!

# 7

# Resources

Campbell, M., Jialal, I. (2022, September 26). *Physiology, Endocrine Hormones*. PubMed; StatPearls Publishing. https://www.ncbi.nlm.ni h.gov/books/NBK538498/

Franziska Spritzler, RD, CDE. (2017, May 15). *12 Natural Ways to Balance Your Hormones*. Healthline; Healthline Media. https://www.healthline.c om/nutrition/balance-hormones

Johnson, J. (2018, December 18). *How to balance hormones naturally: 11 ways*. Www.medicalnewstoday.com. https://www.medicalnewstoday.c om/articles/324031

John Hopkins Medicine. (2019). *Hormones and the Endocrine System*. Johns Hopkins Medicine. https://www.hopkinsmedicine.org/health/ conditions-and-diseases/hormones-and-the-endocrine-system

Li, I. (2016, June). *Nutrition for Seniors*. Delaware Journal of Public Health. https://doi.org/10.32481/djph.2016.06.012

National Institute on Aging. (2022, February 25). *Healthy eating as you age: Know your food groups*. National Institute on Aging. https://www.ni

a.nih.gov/health/healthy-eating-nutrition-and-diet/healthy-eating-you-age-know-your-food-groups

*The basics of an anti-inflammatory diet.* (2024, August 27). Institute for Optimum Nutrition. https://www.ion.ac.uk/news/the-basics-of-an-anti-inflammatory-diet

Zorn, K. (2023, November 16). *The Benefits of Eating an Anti-Inflammatory Diet.* CARESPACE Health+Wellness. https://carespace.health/post/the-benefits-of-eating-an-anti-inflammatory-diet/

Delfin, J., Delfin, J. (2024, August 16). *The Key Role of Physical Activity in Longevity - Welbrook Memory Care.* Welbrook Memory Care. https://www.welbrookmemorycare.com/the-key-role-of-physical-activity-in-longevity/

National Institute on Aging. (2022, June 30). *How can strength training build healthier bodies as we age?* National Institute on Aging. https://www.nia.nih.gov/news/how-can-strength-training-build-healthier-bodies-we-age

Semeco, A. (2021, December 14). *The Top 10 Benefits of Regular Exercise.* Healthline. https://www.healthline.com/nutrition/10-benefits-of-exercise

Warburton, D. E. R., Nicol, C. W., Bredin, S. S. D. (2006, March 14). *Health Benefits of Physical activity: the Evidence.* Canadian Medical Association Journal. https://doi.org/10.1503/cmaj.051351

Askinazi, O. (2023, July 21). *Hormonal insomnia: symptoms, causes, treatments.* Healthline. https://www.healthline.com/health/insomnia/hormonal-insomnia-symptoms

*Comprehensive Guide to Sleep Hygiene.* (2024). Mentally Fit Pro. https://www.mentallyfitpro.com/c/share-a-resource/comprehensive-guide-to-sleep-hygiene

Nowakowski, S., Meers, J., Heimbach, E. (2013, June 30). *Sleep and Women's Health.* Sleep Medicine Research. https://doi.org/10.17241/smr.2013.4.1.1

Suni, E., Singh, A. (2023, December 8). *20 tips for how to sleep better.* Sleep Foundation. https://www.sleepfoundation.org/sleep-hygiene/ healthy-sleep-tips

Mariotti, A. (2015, November 1). *The effects of chronic stress on health: new insights into the molecular mechanisms of brain–body communication.* Future Science OA. https://doi.org/10.4155/fso.15.21

Mayo Clinic Staff. (2023, August 1). *Chronic stress puts your health at risk.* Mayo Clinic; Mayo Foundation for Medical Education and Research. https://www.mayoclinic.org/healthy-lifestyle/stress-management/in -depth/stress/art-20046037

Toussaint, L., Nguyen, Q. A., Roettger, C., Dixon, K., Offenbächer, M., Kohls, N., Hirsch, J., Sirois, F. (2021). *Effectiveness of Progressive Muscle Relaxation, Deep Breathing, and Guided Imagery in Promoting Psychological and Physiological States of Relaxation* (R. Taylor–Piliae, Ed.). Evidence-Based Complementary and Alternative Medicine. https://doi.org/10.115 5/2021/5924040

lifecoachtraining. (2023, July 12). *Exploring the Science Behind the Mind-Body Connection.* Life Coach Certification Online. https://lifecoachtraini ng.co/exploring-the-science-behind-the-mind-body-connection/